NO FILLER · 100% AL[...] FOR LIFE, NOT JUST [...] WILL THANK YOU FOR READING THIS... FOR LIFE! · START BEING A GREAT DAD TODAY! · GOT QUESTIONS? READ ME! · LEARN SOMETHING? TEACH SOMETHING! · IT'S A LONG GAME · TIME TO BE FLEXIBLE · DON'T STOP DATING! · IT'S IN YOU TO BE AN AWESOME DAD · ROUTINE TIME · TIME TO BE AN OPTIMIST · NO FILLER · 100% ALL TRUTH · BEING A DAD IS FOR LIFE, NOT JUST 9 MONTHS · YOUR FAMILY WILL THANK YOU FOR READING THIS... FOR LIFE! · START BEING A GREAT DAD TODAY! · GOT QUESTIONS? READ ME! · LEARN SOMETHING? TEACH SOMETHING! · IT'S A LONG GAME · TIME TO BE FLEXIBLE · DON'T STOP DATING! · IT'S IN YOU TO BE AN AWESOME DAD · ROUTINE TIME · TIME TO BE AN OPTIMIST

Praise for Babies Don't Talk & Truedad

"Being one half of a two-dad family provides a unique perspective to ownership of traditional roles. I would recommend every dad, especially new dads, read this book!"

- Brian

"This was so great for my husband, but also gave me a totally different perspective on so many of those early days. I wish we had this earlier on!"

- Vanessa

"Hey mate, I just wanna say how stoked I was to see you in your field! In a world of so many bullshit instagram coaches and "experts" I couldn't think of anyone more legit doing what you're doing."

- Peter W.

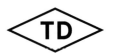

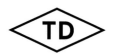

BABIES
DON'T TALK

HONEST INSIGHTS FOR NEW & EXPECTING DADS THAT BUILD A STRONG FOUNDATION FOR FATHERHOOD... I PROMISE.

GRAHAM MECKLING

First published in 2023 by Meck Ventures Ltd.

© Graham Meckling || Meck Ventures Ltd.

The moral rights of the author have been asserted.

Author: Meckling, Graham

Title: Babies Don't Talk: Honest insights for new & expecting dads that build a strong foundation for fatherhood... I promise.

ISBN: 9781738822546

Cover and text design: Tanner Wilson

Dedication

I would like to dedicate this book to each of the following beauties!

Jonesy: there is no doubt that without someone as inspiring as you, I would never have had the fortune of being a dad in a family this full of love, compassion, and teamwork.

You allow me to be the dad I am through your love and support, and I will always know how truly lucky I am to have found you.

Mom and Dad: I knew from a young age that you were both special and the family you created was just as magical. I've learned more from you than you will ever know.

Tanner: None of this happens without you taking an idea and making it into reality. A million thank yous friend.

Weston, Addison, and Glenlivet (my puppy): you are the reason for everything. I love you.

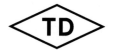

Table of Contents

"This book will make you a more confident dad, not a more insecure one."

–Graham Meckling

01

START THRIVING, NOT SURVIVING

I wonder what's more challenging—the first hundred days of being President or surviving the first hundred days of fatherhood.

If you have a little trouble deciding what to do, there is a phone you can pick up or one of a hundred people ready to help with every detail.

I know that in my early days of fatherhood, I was too busy even to know where my phone was, let alone call for help, and if I did reach someone, they each had completely different instructions, and they certainly didn't have a degree in what they were talking about.

When my wife and I were pregnant, we were handed what seemed like textbooks for what was on the way. I didn't plan on becoming a doctor; just looking for a tip or two for how to change a diaper, what this thing was going to eat, and what I'm supposed to have around the house other than nice cocktail glasses and a few guitars. I didn't want to be overwhelmed by information or have someone make me feel even more insecure by telling me how little I knew...I read three pages.

That's why I'm writing this for you. So you can get a head start on sorting out your new life in less than an hour (depending on how fast you read). I cover what matters most for new and expecting dads: yourself, your partner/relationship, your family, and your child. I've owned a couple of restaurants, like food and drink, play music, and I love my wife. I'm not an obstetrician; I'm not an author...as I write this ;) nor am I the perfect dad (psst... they don't exist)... I'm a guy trying to get through each day with a new life, figuratively and literally.

Even if you put this down after four paragraphs, you should know that every child is unique, and every dad is unique. There is a chance that nothing in this book will work for you and that it ends up a doorstop, but that's ok. Because if that is the case, you may have ruled out one more thing to stop your baby from screaming bloody murder at 2 am.

Read away, friend, and keep your head up!

Life is going to be amazing!

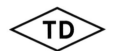

*"Forgive yourself for not having the foresight to know what now
seems so obvious in hindsight."*

–Judy Belmont

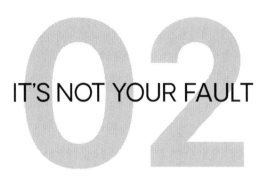

IT'S NOT YOUR FAULT

This book is your starting point.

I keep it simple, honest and concise (just the way we like it) so without further ado, let's crack some eggs and make a family omelette.

All I ever wanted to do was be a dad. Yup! That's it... a dad. Growing up, I thought everything was interesting; Astronaut? Cool. CEO? Cool. Athlete? Cool. Just not as cool as a dad. Because from a young age, I knew I was lucky. I had been blessed with the most magical of gifts, great parents.

They very rarely fought, they hugged all the time, we had family kisses, and I always felt loved. It was magic.

As I grew up, what I envisioned was not just me as a dad with my kids but a family unit. There is no way I am the man I am today without both my mom and dad working as a team to raise their children. Parenting is teamwork, and I had two captains.

BUT the day I saw those two lines on the pregnancy test, I knew there was a massive disconnect between my having all the passion, want, great relationships, friends, family etc..... and the harsh reality that I had virtually no idea of what to do next.

That scared me, made me frustrated, and frankly, I was embarrassed that for all these years of talking about how excited I was for fatherhood, my first day knowing we were going to have a baby was filled with the opposite of the emotions I wanted. Excitement became guilt, and wonder became fear.

How did this happen? How did I end up at this moment? Unfortunately, it's simple. People don't teach the hard stuff. There is a reason people won't tell you what it's like to lose a loved one, to manage money, build a successful long-term relationship, and, yes, to parent. It's simply because it's not easy to teach someone those skills when you yourself have struggled with them.

My dad is the most incredible human on the planet and a fantastic father, but never once did he pull me aside and say, "let me tell you what you really need to know about having a child." We only have one dad. One example to look to, and in many cases no dad at all, for what to do, and just because you can make a baby certainly doesn't mean you are great at raising it.

I never once went for beers with my best friends and talked babies... ever. As men, we grow up sexualizing a vagina and not wanting to talk about a baby coming out of one.

Men just don't grow up with the same support groups as women. Perhaps that's because a watermelon isn't coming out of their penis. If I were going to have a pebble pop out of my penis at some point, I would be talking with every dad I knew about the experience and what precisely that pebble was going to be doing to my body.

Long story short, it's ok. It's not your fault.

Unless you spend ten years studying to become a doctor specializing in pregnancy and childbirth, then take another seven years studying the psychology of relationships and child-raising, it's ok not to know everything.

Every child is unique, every dad is unique, and every relationship is unique. You have time to learn to parent and develop your skills to be great at it.

This book will build a foundation for you to raise a FAMILY on. So let's set you and your new family up for success of the best kind, long-lasting.

"I'm not telling you it will be easy. I am telling you it will be worth it."

-Art Williams

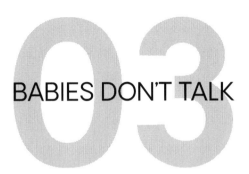

BABIES DON'T TALK

Now that you know it's ok to not know everything lets get to the goods! When I'm asked what my best 'tip' is, I always say the same thing...

"Your baby will not talk to you for two years. Who do you think you'll be talking to every single day? That's right, your partner."

Keeping your relationship strong is the most critical piece of the baby-raising puzzle.

All your baby needs is love, food, sleep, and to be kept clean.

If your fatherhood experience is challenging, it's time for a 30-second hug (See chapter 11), check in with your partner, check in with yourself and reset.

Happy parents = happy baby.

For the longest time, I left this chapter this short and halfway down the chapter list...

I figured some things don't need a lot of filler, examples, or How-to's. They just need to be stated out loud.

But after talking with my wife Michelle, I realize that 'babies don't talk' sums up what this book is about. It's about reframing the dad experience and expectations of fatherhood. How, at this point, dads and partners need this book to be about how your life changes, how your relationship is impacted, and how time, feelings and thoughts all change when you have a baby. AND how all of those have nothing to do with how many ounces of milk to feed a baby, what type of soother is the best, how to hold your baby etc....

As you will read along the way, there will be a lifetime of learning all the medical needs of your child. It can't be crammed into an all-night session the day before your partner goes into labour. There isn't a friend who has all the answers because the questions don't stop coming.

This book will show you a real and true perspective on how to be prepared for the upcoming shift in your life. If you take care of yourself, stay connected with your partner, and stay involved in the process of your new baby, you'll be great... I promise :)

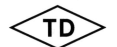

"To thy own self be true."

-Shakespeare

04

DON'T STOP BEING YOU

At your core, you are who you are. I feel the most genuine when I am at my cabin and surrounded by family and memories.

When you are in the midst of the realization that you know so little about something so important as raising a child, it can seem like you are miles away from being what and whom you need to be.

Remember, there is absolutely no such thing as a perfect dad. There is only you and your desire to be great at being a dad.

Take the pressure off of being perfect and put it to the side. There is no hiding who you are from your children. They will know you better than you know yourself. Your baby, from day one, will feel how authentic you are in the energy that you give them.

You simply do not have to change everything about yourself to be a great dad. Embrace the things that make you feel amazing and as always and forever continue to work on the things that you think need improvement.

Love yourself, be genuine, try your best, and you'll be a better dad than you ever thought possible because it's easy to feel like you don't deserve to do the things that define you when you start your fatherhood journey.

Don't let your insecurity make you feel like you don't deserve anything good. Don't let the nasty inside voice say It's not time to play your guitar, read your favourite book, or go for your morning run.

Becoming a dad doesn't mean you stop doing what you love; you're supposed to KEEP doing what you love!

It's doing what you love that defines the best parts of you. It's probably what attracted your partner to you in the first place, and don't forget that your baby will end up knowing you better than you could ever have imagined, so keeping from them the things that make you smile, laugh, and feel good deep down inside would be so unfortunate!

Do the things you love and, if possible, do them with your little one!

A happy dad = a happy baby.

KEEP BELIEVING IN YOURSELF

DON'T LOSE THAT WHICH DEFINES YOU

SCHEDULE SOME 'ME' TIME FOR BOTH PARENTS

"The days are long, but the years are short."

-Gretchen Rubin

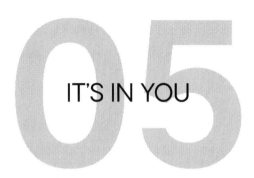

IT'S IN YOU

Ever feel like you are the only one that has gone through something? Transport yourself to the teenage days when it seemed that the whole world just didn't understand what you were feeling.

Next up, parenting! You can feel like you are on an island of loneliness with everyone now out of reach and no one getting just how hard this all is. Well, good news friends! Millions and millions of dads have raised children, and many of those millions have done it without any previous child-raising experience. But how is this possible? How could they have done it without going to school or having years upon years of practice?

I remember Michelle and I decided to take Weston to Mexico when he was only three months old. Of course, like many first-time parents, we made an appointment to see our doctor to discuss all the health challenges this trip would entail.

Does he need shots? Can he be out in the sun? Do we need fancy sunscreen? Can he go into the ocean? Can Michelle eat everything or will it go through the breast milk and make him sick? ..... As we were peppering our Doc with these questions, she had a smirk on her face and finally said, as we were winding down...."Guess what? There are babies in Mexico."

It can't be stressed enough that you'll feel scared to make mistakes. I mean who would want to hurt or make sick this little tiny helpless baby? This is what happens when we let ourselves be overwhelmed by the voice of doubt. The voice tells us that we are just not up to this, or that asking for help is a weakness, or that maybe it's just best to skip what you are planning to do altogether because it's just safer that way.

Remind yourself that many of those millions of dads/partners have done it successfully without training and support. Many of those millions have done it in poverty, alone, or through hardship.

You have the innate ability to parent. Again, you have the innate ability to parent! It's in you to do it and to do it great. Society is great at instilling fear and doubt about our ability to do so many things, but I assure you... you can and will be amazing. All you need is a heaping spoonful of dedication and a cup of commitment, and you'll be great. You are your child's hero from day one. They won't care about your job, how 'cool' you are, or your successes or failures. If you are there and trying, you are winning.

IT'S NORMAL TO BE NERVOUS

YOU HAVE THE STRENGTH TO BE A GREAT DAD REGARDLESS OF THE OBSTACLES

YOU ARE NUMBER ONE TO YOUR BABY FROM DAY ONE

"*Have patience. All things are difficult before they become easy.*"

-Saadi

BUILD PATIENCE TO BUILD SUCCESS

No one will ever blame you for being late if you have a baby... ever. I often joke that every baby gives you a ten-minute window to be late. Many of us are addicted to clocks, timers, deadlines, and lap times. This is one of those benefits of parenting that should be embraced. You can be late and that's ok. It's always ok.

Rushing to be on time usually leads to forgetting something important and having to go back home. Rushing leads to frustration and useless arguments and spats. Rushing leads to amplifying hunger, thirst, and just about everything else.

When the baby arrives, there is a feeling of greater importance on all the little things.

Making it home on time.

Get the milk before it's too hot or too cold

All ten new things just added to your to-do list

Appointment times that can't be missed

Etc...

Leaving the house can be a mission for a team of ten people. Who is in charge of making sure the baby bag is packed? Who is on top of making sure the baby is changed and clean and dressed? Who is packing the car? Who has the backup plan if everything just blows up and you have to come back home halfway to where you are going?

Remember that you have time. Take these moments to practice your patience skills. This is one of those traits that will constantly be tested for the next twenty years.

'Patience is a virtue,' my mom must have said to me a million times over, and she was right. It's not easy and takes time to develop this skill if you don't have it already, so be prepared to have lots of practice time.

PATIENCE WILL BE TESTED
SO BE READY

FIND TIMES THAT ARE
OFTEN RUSHED AND FIND
WAYS TO IMPROVE THEM

PATIENCE TAKES PRACTICE
AND TIME

If Plan A didn't work...the alphabet has twenty-five more letters. Stay cool.

-The Internet

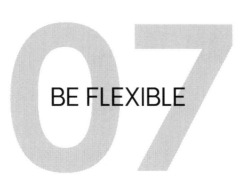

BE FLEXIBLE

The good news is that this chapter is not about touching your toes!

Are you heading out for the first time in months?

Going to see some friends?

Planned a great adventure?

If you are bringing your new baby with you, be prepared to be flexible. It's always good to have a backup plan in case the best strategy gets blown up by the little one because sometimes the baby will decide that the best plan just isn't going to be the one that works.

You might try and be proactive and plan for every circumstance, but if a baby feels like not getting with the program, you don't stand much chance of changing its mind.

But...If you have a fun backup plan...

"Let's put the baby down and play some cards."

"Let's head home and have dual foot rubs."

"Let's get home and just get some extra rest."

You'll take the pressure off everything going perfectly according to plan A.

You will undoubtedly spend much more time at home when your baby arrives, and your house may or may not be set up for being home for extended periods. That's why it's essential to have options to keep you busy when you head back, so you don't go stir-crazy.

Be flexible and have a great night no matter what the baby decides. It can quickly feel that the baby is making decisions when things go awry. They may make the first one, but you can choose the rest.

If you learn to enjoy plan B just as much as plan A it's a win-win.

BOARD GAMES, CARDS, BOOKS AND PUZZLES!

ALWAYS HAVE A FUN BACKUP PLAN

PLANS DON'T HAVE TO WORK OUT PERFECTLY

"Optimism is essential to achievement, and it is also the foundation of courage and true progress."

-Nicolas M. Butler

WHO NEEDS AN UMBRELLA

Fear of the unknown?

Are you dreading a lousy night's sleep?

Are you worried about an adventure?

Unsure if it's enough milk in the bottle?

Time to be an optimist!

It's easy to accept that the day will be hard when you are tired and overwhelmed or to tell yourself that things will not go your way.

That's the tired and pessimistic brain talking, and it can be very persuasive if you let it.

Show up optimistic, and you'll overcome the first hurdle of the day by saying...

"It's ok; I love the rain!"

"I forgot your blanket? Let's use my sweater!"

"You feel like a cry? Well perfect! I feel like a cuddle!"

"Backseat of the car spit up? No worries! It needs a wash!"

When you wake up, think positive and don't let the little things get in the way of your glass being half full.

I remember finding it so challenging to be awake most of the night or to be sound asleep and woken up to take care of a baby at 3 am. Soon enough though, that difficult time became no big deal as your body adjusts and your comfort level rises. Now I can be woken up at any hour in the morning to soothe a child and then fall back asleep in seconds. Without getting grumpy!

It is much easier to say "be optimistic" as I sit at a keyboard typing and not being in your shoes, so remember this: everything changes in the early days of fatherhood and keep your eyes peeled for the tough spots in your new life. When you are confronted by a difficult situation, try adding it to a routine (add prepping your lunch for the next day to your night routine), or perhaps swapping it with your partner (I'll do the grocery shopping if you make the lunch) to help keep you positive. Both your partner and baby will thank you for being an optimist.

Psst...if it's just 'one of those days' and you can't shake off the blues, it's a great time to ask for a 30-second hug!

DON'T FALL INTO A RABBIT HOLE OF PESSIMISM

WORK ON OPTIMISM LIKE EVERYTHING ELSE

WHEN IN DOUBT, ASK FOR A 30-SECOND HUG!

"Feelings are much like waves. We can't stop them from coming, but we can choose which ones to surf."

–Jonatan Martensson

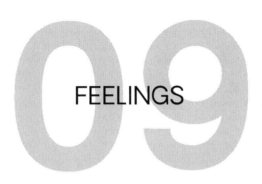

FEELINGS

When you first see your new baby, it's like sticking your finger in an emotional light socket. Your brain is on fire with so many feelings and emotions it can be overwhelming and hard to think straight.

If you are not a big mush ball, never cry at movies, or refuse to listen to a ballad, then heads up... this part will be hard, take practice and time.

For my entire life, before I had children, I never raised my voice, yelled, stomped my feet or got truly angry. I prided myself in my calm nature and positive outlook, but when your baby has been up for hours, and you are running on little sleep, watch out.... There is a new you hiding inside, and your baby is going to bring it out, and it's shocking.

Here is a tip from my business and life coach, Shawn K. Carpenter of The Ollin Group, when asked to describe feelings:

"Learning to properly process your emotions is critical to your well-being and, ultimately, your fulfillment in life. Most people don't feel. They react. This means going much deeper than just the reactionary emotions, as powerful as they may be. It means facing and feeling all that we've been unwilling to face in ourselves, unravelling our unconscious narratives and meeting unmet needs. From there, you can experience the glory, peace, joy, and love that is your essential and true nature."

So when you think some of these thoughts (and you will....)

"I can't handle this!"

"I just don't know what to do"

"I'm leaving"

"I'm an awful father for being so angry at my baby"

Remember to take a deep breath, ask for help, talk to your partner, call a loved one, reach out for help, and most importantly, love yourself and don't give up.

TIME TO GET TO KNOW
YOUR FEELINGS

THE BETTER YOU
UNDERSTAND YOU THE
BETTER

ASK FOR HELP AND ASK FOR
HUGS

"The best thing to spend on your relationship is time, conversation, understanding, and honesty."

-Anonymous

DON'T STOP DATING

Sounds simple, doesn't it?

Let us assume that there was a reason you and your partner decided to bring a new life into the one you are currently living... Love!

It's powerful and beautiful but can be put to the test when the baby comes. You'll find your head spinning, mama will be in pain, you'll be exhausted from the last few weeks of build-up before the baby arrived, still working, not sleeping, and the list goes on. It cannot be stated enough how important it is to keep the connection between you and your partner strong right from the start. This is what 'building a foundation' is all about. Don't wait for the relationship to get rough before you start putting in the work, especially when all you need to do is keep doing what made you fall in love in the first place!

Taking the time to be together will keep you connected to each other. This may be hard to do depending on your partner's recovery from delivery, but if possible, I recommend once every two weeks to spend some alone time at a minimum. Remember that a date can be as small as having a neighbour come over while the baby is napping for a ten-minute walk around the block to having grandparents or friends watch the little one so you can grab a coffee or a beer and sparkling water date :)

It's so easy to get into the wrong new roles once the baby arrives if you are not prepared. Many dads recall how they felt so insecure around mom and baby that it felt better to be 'at the office' or 'getting groceries' because they felt they were contributing somewhere, even if it wasn't at home.

Of course, the mom is still at home with the baby and feeling the weight and responsibility of being the one to do everything, and then before you know it, the dreaded 'me vs. you' scale comes out....

Dad "I have been out all day running errands, getting the food and diapers!"

Mom "Well, I am breastfeeding and keeping the house clean!"

How quickly we can move from the excitement of a baby to tired, frustrated, angry, and resentful. This is why spending time with each other to focus on taking a deep breath, laugh, or nap is essential. Keeping the emotional connection strong will help keep your lines of communication positive and allow you to stay on top of how you are both doing. Empathy and caring for each other are foundational components for building your family.

DON'T STOP WORKING ON YOUR RELATIONSHIP

PLAN YOUR DATE NIGHTS IN YOUR NEW LIFE SCHEDULE

DATES CAN BE SMALL OR BIG... JUST MAKE SURE YOU HAVE THEM!

"*I have learned that there is more power in a good strong hug than in a thousand meaningful words.*"

-Ann Hood

THIRTY-SECOND HUGS

Knowing how feeling tired, exhausted, and on edge can translate into your daily life is crucial. We need to recognize how we speak and communicate with our partners, not only when things are going great, and we are filled with enthusiasm, but even more critically when we are low on juice and our voice sends out the wrong message and with the wrong intent.

No matter how much you prepare to be the best partner and how many vows you make about talking and listening with empathy and compassion, you will have challenging moments.

It's usually over the same things you 'fought' about before the baby. These little scraps filled with annoyance have become full tilt and filled with anger. So how do we put the brakes on once the car has started rolling down the street?

HUG... and do it for 30 seconds.

This is one that both partners need to be prepared for. If someone is genuinely hurt and angry, it can be challenging to accept a hug. Use this method by asking for a deep breath for you and your partner. Next, acknowledge that the tension is more than likely due to exhaustion and not what is being argued about. Finally, ask for 'the hug' and don't let go.

Take ten seconds to let the tension subside, ten seconds to say I'm sorry, and ten seconds to squeeze a little tighter and let it all go.

Finish this moment by revisiting the reason for the argument in calm voices and with a clear perspective.

Let the hug do its job and bring you both back to even.

SLOW DOWN THE TENSION

RECOGNIZE THE REAL
REASON FOR SMALL
PROBLEMS

ASK FOR A HUG TO
CONNECT AND CHILL

"Tell me, and I forget. Teach me, and I remember. Involve me, and I learn."

–Benjamin Franklin

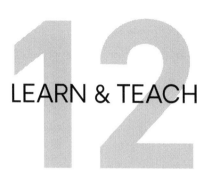

LEARN & TEACH

Nothing saddens me more then when I hear a parent say to the other in a condescending tone, "That's not how you do it. Let me." This is one of those lines that can cut to the core of someone trying so hard to be a great involved partner, especially through the battle of insecurity or doubt.

If this is both of your first times having a baby, you'll both be fortunate to have so many things to learn and witness. It's going to be impossible to keep track of each time you say "that's amazing!" or "I can't believe that trick worked!" or "I'll never do that again!". Many of these new baby puzzle pieces you'll discover while your partner is away.

Make these learning moments a moment for two. Remember how both of you are probably feeling insecure about your newborn knowledge and use these moments to make each other better parents. Build your knowledge puzzle together and watch the picture come into focus faster and with more clarity.

You'll find that you're learning curve will be cut in half with a daily 'what did you learn?' conversation. You'll be connecting with each other and your baby simultaneously through the sharing of information. This can apply to just about everything in the first hundred days. Since your baby has never experienced anything at all it will take time to see if some things work long-term or if they are just a short-term win.

Your little one might like the cool breeze one day and then cry the next time, or love a warm bath and then fuss if it's warm the next. The key is to share what you notice. Something little to you could be the answer to a long-term puzzle piece. Or simply, if you and your partner are trying different solutions, it will be conflicting to the little one and make the breakthroughs farther apart.

Your relationship with your partner evolves. Your relationship with your baby evolves. Your relationship with your family evolves. When something works, keep at it. It may last for a few weeks; like when I would make little circles between Weston's eyes with my thumb to help him fall asleep, or it may last five minutes; like when Addison stopped crying when I played her guitar :)

The key is to never stop sharing information to make parenting easier and more effective. Share it all so your partner shares something with you that will help the little one sleep when you need it most.

SUPPORT YOUR PARTNER AT ALL TIMES

REMEMBER TO SPEED UP THE LEARNING CURVE THROUGH COMMUNICATION

BE A TEACHER NOT A KEEPER OF NEW BABY INFORMATION

A problem shared is a problem halved

-Proverb

TAKE IT OFF YOUR SHOULDERS

A dad's insecurity and lack of baby knowledge can manifest themselves in several ways. One of the most distressing is how it can put the pressure to raise the new baby solely on the mom's shoulders.

Many moms find themselves trying to raise the baby and train the dad. They see their partner moving further away from their daily responsibilities and struggling to find out where they fit in, but it doesn't have to be this way.

If we keep our relationship strong and our daily lines of communication strong and open, we will keep parenting a partnership.

The 'jobs' are not delegated as mine and yours but as 'ours.' Tell your partner that you are there not just to support but lead, and if there are things that need to be done, you are willing to learn how and take the boulder of the responsibility off their shoulders.

Not every family has to fit into the 1950s model of mom at home and dad at work. That dynamic has shifted for so many. Whether you have a two-mom family, two-dad family, stay-at-home dad etc.. choosing who needs to do which role and each chore just needs to be discussed.

The tasks and roles can change daily, weekly, monthly or by the hour. Be open to learning new skills and you'll both become powerhouse parents.

IT'S YOUR PARTNER'S FIRST TIME WITH A NEW BABY TOO!

EVERY SITUATION IS UNIQUE SO FIND WAYS THAT HELP SUPPORT YOUR PARTNER

LEARN NEW SKILLS IN ADVANCE FOR BABY

Grace is understanding, compassion, and says, "It's ok. We are in this together."

-Graham Meckling

14
GRACE – GIVE IT AND GET IT

Babies don't have jobs, hundreds of personal and professional relationships, full schedules, or a complicated past! They just want a full tummy, a clean bottom, and some sleep with mom or dad.

And good news! No one ever said... When I was a baby, I remember my dad saying, "I'm having a hard time with this!" Or "Why won't you just stop crying?!"

You will make tons of mistakes, which is 100% normal and 100% expected!

You will overfeed your baby, and they'll throw it back up!... You'll underfeed your baby, and they'll cry because it's too late to feed them now!... You'll wake them up by accident; you'll try and put them down when they want to be awake!.. You'll check a bum to see if it needs changing, and the minute you've cleaned it and wrapped them back up, they'll poop, and you won't notice it, then wonder why they keep crying only to notice they've now got diaper rash.

I remember telling Michelle that one of us is going to drop the baby or hurt the baby by accident and whoever does it gets a massive hug because they are going to feel awful!

Embrace the mistakes and know that mistakes are a part of parenting. Embrace the fact that you have time before the baby starts telling all its baby friends about that time the milk was too hot or the windows were left open a crack and it was freezing overnight.

Remember that trying is winning!

YOU WILL MAKE MISTAKES, AND THAT IS PART OF THE PROCESS

BE READY TO SAY, "IT'S OK." BECAUSE AN 'OOPS' IS GOING TO HAPPEN TO YOU

BABIES DON'T RAT YOU OUT

"It's the little things in life."

-Every mom

SET THEM UP FOR SUCCESS

Got five minutes? Give five minutes!

This is one of those things that stuck like glue from my restauranteur days. The day team sets up the night team and vice versa. It's always hard to start your shift if you have to spend the first part getting set up.

When it comes to parenting, this one feels like magic. If you find yourself with a free five minutes...

Stock up the baby bag!
Fold some laundry!
Do some dishes!
Prep a meal!
Write a love note!

It's the little things, isn't it, that make us feel special? In the first few months, it goes so far to get and give a little love.

You'll both be low on juice, and taking a few moments to show your partner that you are both on the same team and going through the same emotions will tremendously impact the day-to-day early stages of parenting.

In the first few months, you can really start to feel like ships in the wind, just high-fiving each other on the way by to the next step in the day. A great move is to have a few sticky notes handy, dry-erase board or chalkboard paint wall to quickly and easily leave a 'hi' or 'love note'.

Communication is key. Making it easy to do it? It's a win. Also, this is a great way to bring love and energy back your way. Not only will it feel good to give some positivity, but it will also feel great getting some in return.

Set up your partner for success, and you'll simultaneously set up your family for success.

FIND SOME SNEAKY AND
FUN WAYS TO HELP OUT

SURPRISE SUPPORT IS
BEAUTIFUL

LITTLE MOMENTS HAVE A
BIG IMPACT

"Before anything else, preparation is the key to success."

-Alexander Graham Bell

16

BOUNDARIES & EXPECTATIONS

Do you think you are excited to meet your new baby? Well, guess what... your parents are even more excited! They have been waiting for twenty to thirty years for the grandkids to come along and, in many cases, want nothing more than to be as involved as possible.

Remember that our parent's generation was raised with moms supposed to be at home raising kids and dads supposed to be at work. It was not cool for a man to ask for help, admit his insecurities, and most certainly not be required to be an involved dad from day one.

Can you imagine how badly they must want their babies (that means you) not to go through what they went through? If you had next to zero support, had no training, and went through a war with your babies and partner, you would do anything to save your children the same heartache.

Parents might tell you something along the lines of...

"Trust me; this is how you hold them."

"The best way to have them sleep is this routine."

"I know what to do."

"This worked for you, so it must work for your baby."

These all come from the same place of love, but it's essential to know that YOU are the expert on your baby. It's your choice to do what you feel is suitable for the little one. It can be tricky and sensitive to manage family, but establishing boundaries and expectations from the beginning is the best way to go.

Now, remember that all people and families have unique situations and needs. You will want your family and friends to be there for you 100%, so this is not a recommendation to keep family away but to keep control of your household in the beginning days of the baby's life. You want parents and friends to know they are encouraged to make parenting suggestions, but at the end of the day, they also know that you and your partner are the ones making the final decisions.

Schedule the first week of the baby at home. Let family and friends know when you'd like them to come over, what they can bring (food, food, and food), and when you'd like them to leave.

"It would be great to see you! Please come by Monday at 1 pm and stay till 2 pm. That would be best. Can't wait to have you visit!"

PLAN YOUR FAMILY TIME IN ADVANCE

CHOOSE A START TIME AND AN END TIME FOR VISITS

REMEMBER HOW IMPORTANT THE BABY IS TO EVERYONE ELSE AS WELL

"*A man's friendships are one of the best measures of his worth*"

-Charles Darwin

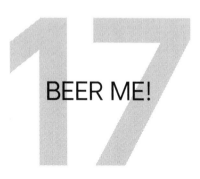

BEER ME!

Michelle and I were social butterflies, to say the least before we had our firstborn, Weston. I owned an award-winning restaurant here in Victoria B.C., and when we weren't hosting friends there, it seemed there was always a steady flow of afternoon bar-b-ques, spot prawn boil-ups, or late night cocktails at our place.

Fast forward to Weston being in the picture, and our house felt like a ghost town from 6 pm onwards.

As many first-time parents tend to do, we watched the T.V. with the volume at two, talked in whispers, and found ourselves saying "shhhh!" constantly.

It was certainly a lifestyle adjustment and not just for us but for our friends. I now had this beautiful baby boy to hold and kiss and play with, and going out for drinks or hosting a big party at our place seemed to be the last thing on my mind.

Keep calling your friends. You'll need them.

I always say to be aware of your own personal social situation for the first three months of having a baby. You might be a dad who handles it with no problem, finds it total madness, or somewhere in the middle. The key is not to try and have the same social life and home life right away.

Let yourself adjust to the new routines in your life, and let your friends adjust to them as well. Make your priority supporting your partner and building your new family foundations first but let your friends know you are thinking of them. When it works, invite them for visits or pop by with the baby. You'll start to develop the balance of being social with your new home life before you know it.

Psst... if you plan on having more than a few drinks make sure you plan on having everything set up for your partner for the day after.

Breakfast prepped? Check!
Laundry done? Check!
All errands done? Check!
Happy partner? Check!

DON'T LOSE CONTACT WITH FRIENDS AND FAMILY

TAKE TIME TO BUILD YOUR NEW FOUNDATIONS

PLAN AHEAD IF YOU PLAN ON BEING OUT LATE

"Patience is a virtue."

-William Langland

18
WELCOME TO THE BACKSEAT

Are you used to being the centre of attention? Well, get used to riding in the backseat for a while :)

It is an odd feeling to be said hello to last, if at all, when you have a new baby. Someone will come over and say immediately, "where is that beautiful little baby?!" ...and run straight past you.

It's hard to blame them, isn't it? If you bought a brand new Ferrari, chances are when you had friends over, that shiny new car would be the first thing they would want to talk about, look at, and play with.

Be ready to be selfless and have patience when it comes to the attention rankings. You'll get your hugs and hellos in due time, but it will be an extra few minutes from now on.

It's going to feel natural to want to whine a bit. After all, you are the one who bought the Ferrari and is putting in all the work and sleepless nights to keep it looking and running top-notch. Now you have to give the keys to everyone who comes over and jump in the backseat while they take it for a joy ride (then pass it back as soon as it poops).

Don't hold it against the baby. It's not the little one's fault that it's new, cute, and is somehow cooler than you already. It's ok. Your family and friends still love you, even if they forget to say it :)

SHARE IN THE EXCITEMENT OF THE BABY

DON'T BLAME THE BABY

"Taking care of yourself doesn't mean me first. It means me too."

-L.R. Knost

19

THE AIRPLANE METHOD

There is a reason they tell you to put on the oxygen mask first and your child second. It's so much more difficult to take care of the needs of your baby if you are frazzled. If you aren't thinking clearly it's not going to get any easier to do anything. You need to make sure you are as happy and positive as possible in all situations to transfer that energy to your little one.

If you are hungry and the baby is crying? Take a breath, put the baby safely in the crib, and eat. If you are exhausted and frustrated and the baby needs you? Take five minutes to calm yourself down and come back better. It's interesting that so many of us believe we need to suffer to feel a sense of accomplishment. That the only way to achieve our goal is by having someone or something inflict pain upon us so that when we finally reach the destination or have a victory we know it by the scars that we got along the way. You can hear it in the comments that one dad will say about another dad when they are at a distance and struggling with a crying baby or a difficult situation.

"Good luck buddy! That's totally the wrong thing to do. Watch this guy suffer!" Or... "Oh, that guy is in for it! He has no idea what he's doing."

Here is one of the moments in my parenting journey that sent me on the path to writing this book:

I remember when it was my turn to take Weston while Michelle got some sleep. It was probably 3 am or so and I rolled out of a deep sleep to head across the hall and do some baby soothing.

It just so happened that Weston felt like crying...and the kind of baby cry that seeps into your bones and blurs everything you've ever known or felt. Like it's only this moment, and it's only this crying you can think of. Looks like it's time to suffer. I tried all of the moves that had worked in the past. The loaf of bread carry and rock, the over-the-shoulder back rub, the white noise giraffe, singing songs, and all the time....suffering.

I spent 30 minutes feeling my anxiety meter climb...then climb some more...

It was then I realized it's airplane method time. I put Weston back in his crib, went to my drawer and found a pair of earplugs, and jammed one in the ear on the side Weston was crying. When I picked him back up, I instantly felt better. I went from the verge of a breakdown to almost giggling at how silly I was for forgetting to take care of myself. There was no nobility in suffering when all it took was a little piece of foam in my ear to have my body calm down, my heartbeat settle, and a smile on my face. Weston was asleep five minutes later. He could feel my energy and matched it.

MAKE SURE YOU TAKE CARE
OF YOURSELF AND WHAT
YOU NEED TOO

PUT YOURSELF IN THE
POSITION TO BEST TAKE
CARE OF YOUR FAMILY

BABIES FEED OFF YOUR
ENERGY SO PAY ATTENTION
TO IT

"I've learned that the long game is the shortcut."

-Richie Norton

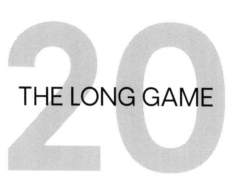

THE LONG GAME

Parenting is a long game and not a short one. There is a great expression that says 'long days and short years'. Just hang in there, and you'll see the results. You will have more wins than failures and although It's easy to beat yourself up for a mistake that happened at that moment, you must remember that you have years to build your skills and time to develop the proper habits for success.

From the day you see the positive pregnancy test, everything will be attached to a time.

How many months along are you?

How many months is the baby?

What is bedtime, milk time, nap time?

What time is my turn?

How long do I heat the milk?

How long is the baby napping for?

How long should the baby be napping?

As a boy growing up my favourite thing to do was play catch with my dad in our back lane. Those hours were the highlight of my youth when I reminisce about back in the day. That was when we chatted about nothing and everything. To me, that was a father-and-son relationship. It wasn't complicated or difficult and didn't take my dad years of study and hardship to do.

I'll never forget being in the midst of a diaper change with Weston and thinking that my dream of playing catch with my son was miles away, like an almost impossible amount of time away from this moment here and now till then.

There will feel a real pressure to know everything and know it yesterday. You don't want to look like this is your first rodeo, but it's painfully obvious it is.

You'll forget to do a hundred important things. You'll make a thousand mistakes.

You will drop the baby.

You will forget to buckle the baby up.

You will yell at the baby.

You will forget to feed the baby.

All of this and more will happen.

You can not be perfect at being a dad because perfection and parenting do not go together. All you need to strive for is being committed to being great. That means putting in the effort day in and day out.

Your version of 'playing catch' will be here before you know it. That impossible amount of time is actually an instant. Take a thousand deep breaths and savour the moments with your baby. Savour the cries and diapers. Savour the late nights and fussing. Savour the time you get to care for your partner and be the caregiver for your family.

It's going to fly by faster than a thought because the baby days are just that. A quick year and then it's off to toddler land and beyond.

Be a sponge and soak up the experience and remind yourself daily or even hourly that it's a long game until your baby says its first word, or feeding itself, or throws a baseball. You have time to be the dad and partner you want and need to be.

YOU WILL HAVE TIME TO
MAKE MISTAKES AND
LEARN

IT'S A LONG GAME SO
BE PATIENT AND STAY
INVOLVED

WORK TOWARDS YOUR
LONG-TERM DAD GOALS

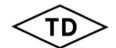

"Your routine is freedom in disguise."

-Graham Meckling

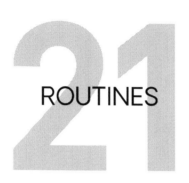

ROUTINES

When the little one arrives in this world, you'll find your sanity through the structure and stability of routines. It may sound like you now have so many new responsibilities and obligations, but you'll soon realize that these routines give you peace of mind and freedom. Raising a baby is hard to do on a whim! Your baby will need you to remember the little things to keep them alive and thriving.

Feeding routine? Check
Leaving the house routine? Check
Bedtime routine? Check

These routines build a calmness in your baby; the more you stick with them, the more your baby knows what's happening and gets with the program. You'll find this especially important for sleep training and meal time. Here is an example of the bedtime routine Michelle and I used for Weston:

1. Bath time
2. Post-bath coconut oil massage
3. A slow walk around the house turning off or down the lights
4. Read books
5. Put on music or white noise
6. Feed
7. Lay baby in the crib, slowly walk out, and cross your fingers :)

Also, the routines will allow you to feel comfortable having the baby on your own and keep your partner and you on the same page. Think of the routines as instructions for raising your baby. Instead of getting a drill and a screwdriver, it's running a bath and warming up the milk.

Each of these steps keeps you involved, keeps you on track, and keeps the baby in the loop for what's happening next. This builds trust and comfort in your little one and creates confidence in yourself and your abilities.

Make sure to write down all of your routines and keep them handy, as they are great for reference when it's date night, and someone is coming over to watch the baby.

You will keep adding to them as the days go by as you see what steps work and which don't.

They will be a working document for the next ten years.

ORGANIZE YOUR TIME TO CREATE YOUR TIME

START WITH MORNING, BEDTIME, AND MEALTIME ROUTINES

A ROUTINE IS A COMMUNICATION AND TEACHING TOOL BETWEEN PARTNERS AND BABY

"Baby girls are like flowers that are forever in bloom."

-Anon

22

BABY GIRLS AND VAGINAS

Why are the early days of pregnancy and fatherhood so hard?

You are faced with many different perspectives and learning curves that can make you feel off kilter. Then...

IT'S A GIRL!

If you are nervous about becoming a dad, I'm guessing you'll be a tad bit anxious about having a girl, but here is some good news.

Most of us men had to try extremely hard to have a woman show some interest in us, let alone fall in love with us enough and commit to spending a lifetime together and whoa... enough to have a baby that is half them and half us.

If you have a daughter, you'll experience having a little lady love you unconditionally from the get-go! That's right! It doesn't matter if you have a pot belly, if you are terrible at math, if you can't hold a tune in a bucket, or stink at all things sports.

You start from the beginning as her all-time favourite dad!

I was and continue to be amazed at the power and strength in a girl as small as my two-year-old. From the beginning, she's got more innate ability and confidence than I feel I've ever had.

I know my Addison will teach me so much about why a woman is who she is, and it will be an honour to empower her and set an example for her for years to come.

You'll also be hearing the word 'vagina' a LOT over the year of pregnancy and birth, especially if you are lucky enough to have a daughter.

As men grow up, we never really take time to get comfortable with the word or learn about it.

When you are a child, the word makes you giggle.
When you're a teen, it 'grosses' you out.
When you're in your 20s, you call it anything but a vagina.

As men growing up, a vagina is something we sexualize, not normalize. But as a dad, you need to understand it.

Get ready to learn how it works and why, so you can help support your partner and help raise a daughter.

ASKING QUESTIONS MAKES YOU A BETTER DAD

SUPPORTING YOUR DAUGHTER STARTS FROM DAY ONE

BE READY TO RAISE A DAUGHTER WITH THE RIGHT INFORMATION

"The man who has confidence in himself, wins the confidence of others."

-Hasidic proverb

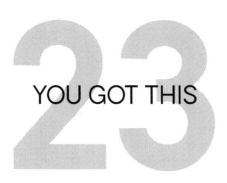

YOU GOT THIS

As you get closer and closer to the day you welcome your baby into this world, remember that you can do this, that millions have done it before you, and that your level of involvement is how you grade your ability as a dad.

It's ok to feel like you'll never get to the top of the information mountain because it never stops growing, just like you, your child, and your relationships. You can only build confidence in your ability one day at a time so start today. Dive in and stay involved. Show your partner that you have the confidence to be a great parent, and not only can they lean on you, but you'll also be confident enough to know when to lean on them.

No one will give you a report card on how 'good or bad' you are as a parent. Perfection is not a term attached to fatherhood because there simply is no standard to look to. You only need to look at the effort and love you pour into your partner, yourself and your baby to determine your success.

Everyone will end up parenting in their own way because we all have unique situations, cultures, and are unique in our upbringing and sense of self.

Give yourself time to become the parent you want to be and grace for when you, or your partner, inevitably make mistakes.

Struggles will come, challenging situations will show up at the worst moments, you may yell, or scream, or feel terrible, and more but know that the moments you'll remember the most will be the kisses, the hugs, the growth of your relationship through communication and empathy, and thanks of your children for working hard at being the best dad you can be.

Welcome to the wonderful world of fatherhood!

YOU GOT THIS!!!

About The Author

Graham Meckling is a proud husband, father and friend. He is an award-winning restauranteur and lives a life dedicated to bringing positivity and love into the world.

He is devoted to teaching dads and partners the honest and true realities of bringing a baby into the world and believes that through education and awareness of what's to come, families will be stronger, last the test of time, and can be filled with passion and commitment.

When not talking fatherhood and babies, you'll find him playing music, throwing a baseball, and hugging whomever gets too close ;)

To get in contact, email him at graham@truedad.ca

On the next page you'll find the Truedad Fridge List ©

Please tear it out and keep it on your fridge to help keep you connected to your goals of staying involved and being a great dad and partner!

Notes

truedad

Plan a date night minimum once every two weeks. Happy parents = happy baby.

Learn something new about baby? Teach your partner and get better together.

Feeling tired, upset, lonely, frustrated? Call for a 30 second hug... longer hugs are welcome!

Don't rush and build your patience skills. It's ok to be late if you have a baby, always.

Long game! You have time to be a great parent so allow each other to make mistakes and give each other grace.

Set your partner and yourself up for success! Got five minutes? Give five minutes!

Don't put it on your shoulders. It takes a village so support support support!

Plan your family and friend visits so you can prepare for them and control your time.

You have the innate ability to be an awesome parent. You can and will be great by staying involved.

TRUEDAD.CA

In honor of:

-Dennis Meckling

To me, you are perfect.

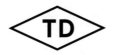